Medicinal Herbs and Herbal Remedies

Herbs You Must Have for Health and Healing

Table of Contents

Introduction

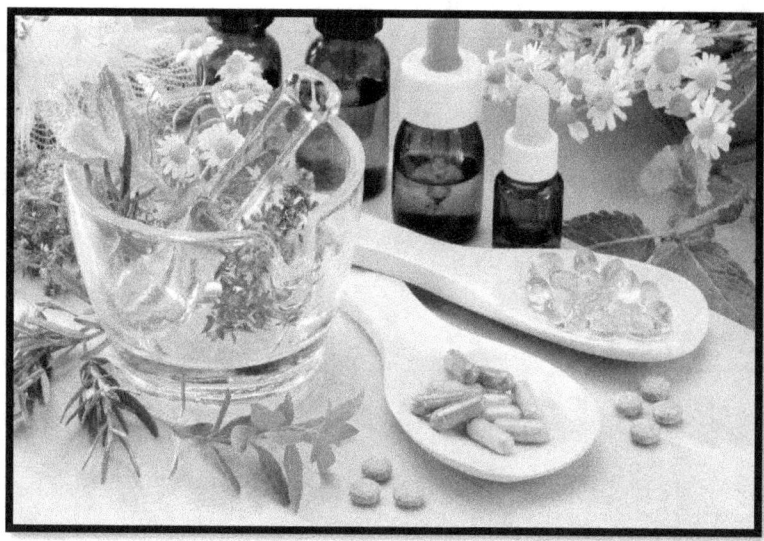

When someone in your family comes down with a cold, what is the first thing you do? You probably run to the drug store for an over-the-counter remedy. What you may not realize is that, in doing so, you may be putting harmful ingredients into your loved one's body that may end up doing more harm than good. If you want to treat common illnesses in a healthy and all-natural way, then consider making your own herbal remedies. In this book, you will find an overview of the benefits of herbal remedies as well as a list of some of the top medicinal herbs. You will also receive a collection of natural herbal remedies to use in treating yourself and your family members.

Medicinal Herb Profiles

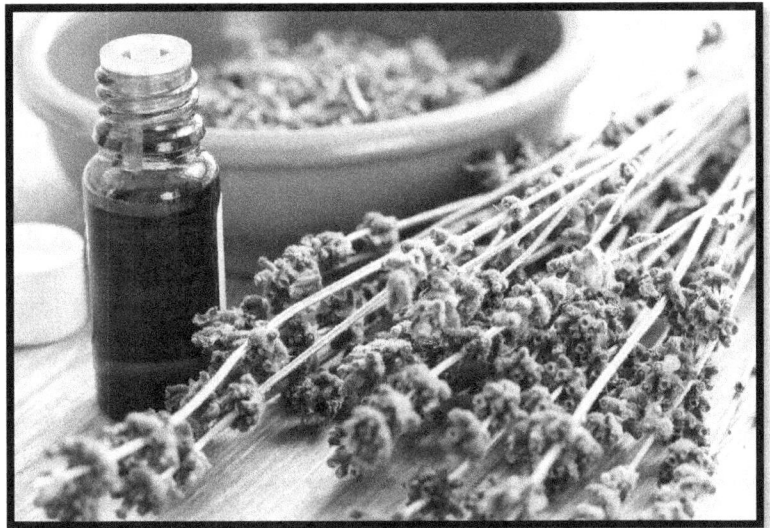

There are hundreds, even thousands of different types of natural herbs that have been used by humans over the centuries. Many of these herbs provide powerful medicinal benefits that are still being used today. <u>Below you will find a list of some of the most commonly used herbs as well as a brief overview of their uses</u>:

Blackberry (*Rubus villosus*) – The leaves, root and bark of the blackberry plant are commonly used to treat diarrhea, dysentery, hemorrhoids, and sore throat.

Calendula (*Calendula officinalis*) – The most valuable parts of the calendula plant are the flowers and essential oils – they can be used to heal wounds, reduce inflammation, to treat acne and to cure thrush.

Cayenne (*Capsicum annuum*) – Cayenne pepper is commonly used as a culinary spice, but the fruit of the plant can be used to treat arthritis, to strengthen digestion, as a heart tonic and to prevent peptic ulcers.

Comfrey (*Symphytum officinale*) – The leaves and roots of the comfrey plant have astringent and expectorant properties – they can be used to treat burns, insect bites, wounds and other skin irritation. It can also heal ulcers and sooth sore throat/cough.

Chamomile (*Matricaria recutita*) – The flowers of the chamomile plant are most commonly used, though the essential oil is powerful as well. Chamomile is typically used as a sleep aid and as a treatment for anxiety, burns, abdominal cramps and other digestive problems.

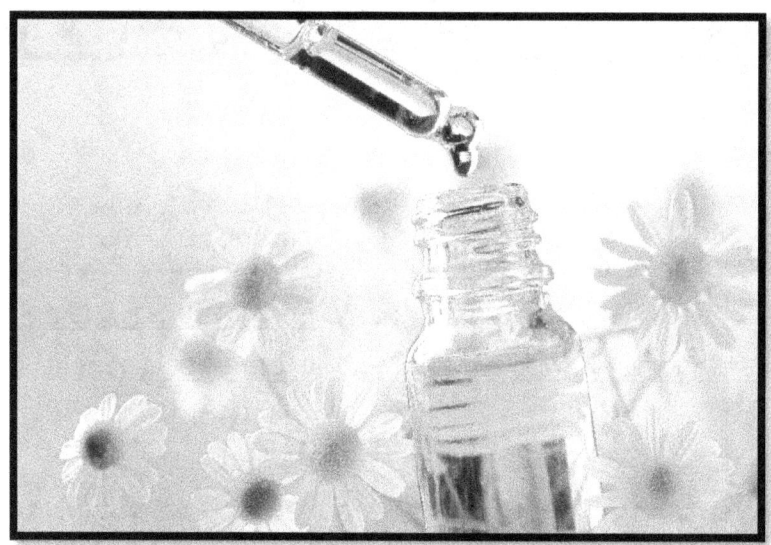

1: Chamomile Essential Oil

Dandelion (*Taraxacum officinale*) – The root of the dandelion plant has powerful diuretic and stomachic properties. It has been used to stimulate digestion, to treat acne and as a natural diuretic.

Echinacea (*Echinacea purpurea*) – The most commonly used part of the Echinacea plant is the root, though the stems and flowers can be used as well. This herb is used to boost the immune system and treat colds, sore throat, sinus infection and yeast infection. It can also be applied topically to treat insect bites and hives.

Fennel (*Foeniculum vulgare*) – The seeds of the fennel plant are the most powerful, though the leaves, roots and essential oil can also be used to treat congestion and cough. The most common use for fennel, however, is as a digestive aid to relieve cramps, gas and bloating.

Goldenseal (*Hydrastis canadensis*) – The root of the goldenseal plant has powerful antifungal, antiviral and immunostimulant properties. This herb can be used to treat sinus infections, congestion, sore throat, diarrhea, ulcers and cuts/wounds.

Ginger (*Zingiber officinalis*) – Commonly used for culinary purposes, ginger root can also be used medicinally to treat nausea, arthritis, abdominal cramps, colds, flu and digestive problems.

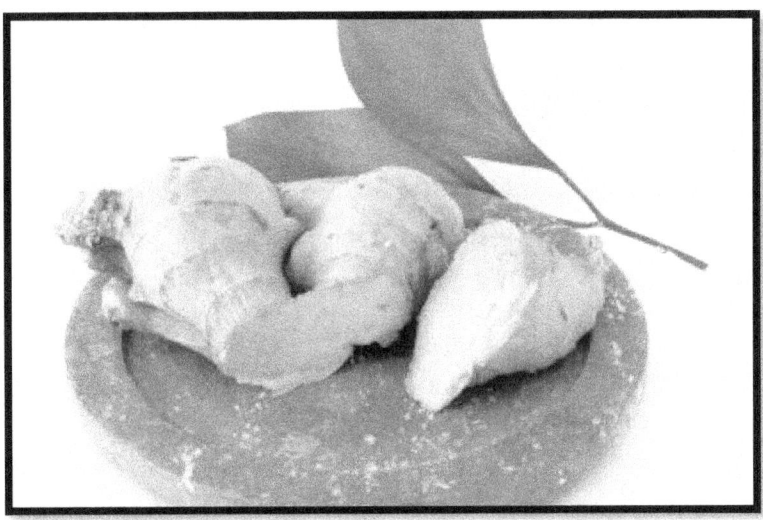

2: Ginger Root

Hawthorn (*Crataegus oxyacanthus*) – The flowers, leaves and berries of the hawthorn plant can be used as a tonic for heart problems and as both a sleep aid and a digestive aid. The flowers and berries can also treat sore throat.

Marshmallow (*Althaea officinalis*) – The root of the marshmallow plant is commonly used as a mucilage – it helps to sooth the throat inside and out as a treatment for congestion, sore throat and cough. It can also be used to treat stomach ulcers and UTI.

Mugwort (*Artemisia vulgaris*) – The leaves and roots of the mugwort plant can be used by women to treat amenorrhea or as a digestive stimulant. It also acts as a mild sedative and can help to ease stress and anxiety.

Mullein (*Verbascum spp.*) – The leaves, flowers and roots of the mullein plant have been used to treat earache, sore throat, coughing and rheumatism. It is also a popular ingredient in tea used to help the lungs recover from smoke damage.

Nettle (*Urtica spp.*) – The leaves and stems of the nettle plant contain natural antihistamines which are helpful in treating allergies and sinus problems. This herb can also be used to treat gout, arthritis and osteoporosis/bone loss.

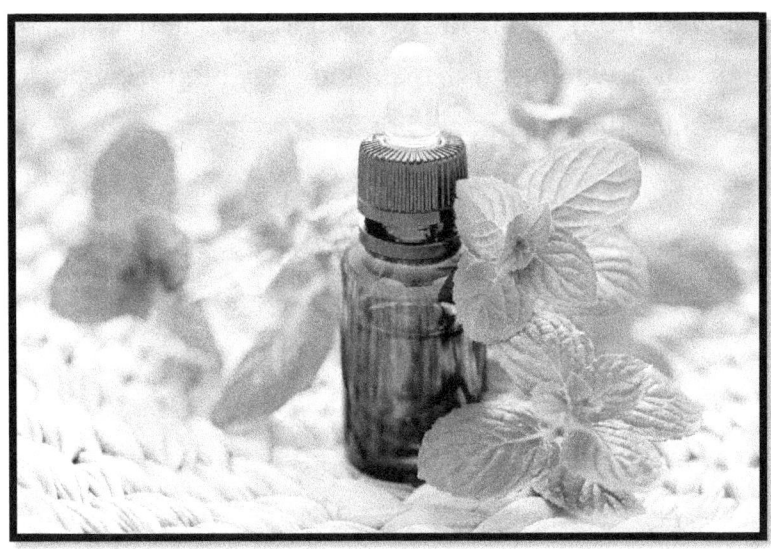

3: Peppermint Essential Oil

Peppermint (*Mentha piperita*) – The leaves of the peppermint plant provide antispasmodic, analgesic, an astringent properties – they can be used to calm nausea, prevent gas/bloating and as a treatment for cold, flu, congestion and headache.

St. John's Wort (*Hypericum perforatum*) – The flowers of the St. John's Wort herb are primarily used as a treatment for depression and anxiety, but they can also be used to treat incontinence, flue, and pain associated with arthritis, PMS and fibromyalgia.

Valerian (*Valeriana officinalis*) – Valerian root is one of the most powerful herbal sedatives and it is commonly used to treat insomnia, anxiety and muscle cramps. When used with hawthorn, it also has a tonic effect on the heart.

Willow Bark (*Salix alba*) – Willow bark has long been used as a treatment for pain and fever – when taken in tea, it acts in a similar way to aspirin for the reduction of pain, fever and inflammation – it can also help prevent heart attack.

Yarrow (*Achillea millefolium*) – Yarrow is known for its astringent properties and is commonly used to disinfect wounds and to staunch bleeding. This herb can also help to reduce fever and expel toxins during a cold or flu.

Benefits of Herbal Remedies

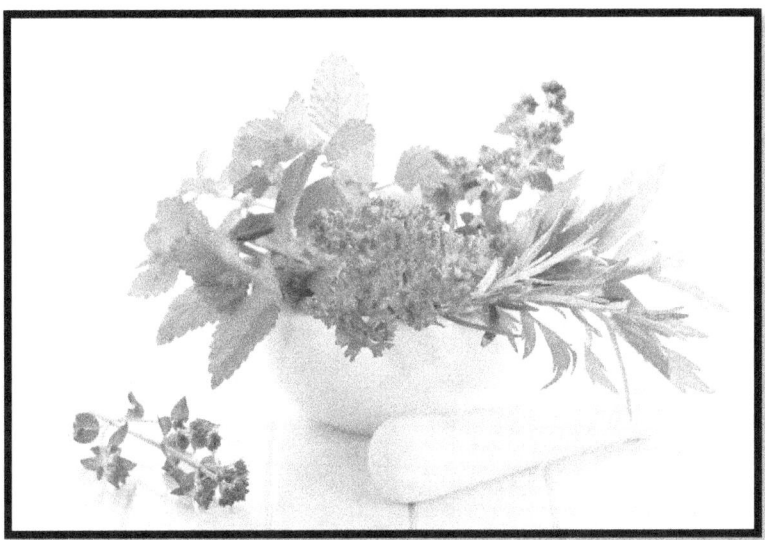

When it comes to treating your loved ones for common illnesses, why would you use something made with artificial ingredients that could end up doing more harm than good? Humans have been using medicinal herbs for centuries in traditional medicine, so why shouldn't you? It is true that there are both disadvantages and advantages for using herbal remedies as an alternative to over-the-counter drugs and medicine, but you will likely find that the good outweighs the bad. <u>Below you will find a list of benefits associated with using herbal remedies</u>:

1. When using herbal remedies, you know what ingredients are being used and how they are likely to affect your body.

2. Herbal remedies have a much lower risk of side effects and they are typically tolerated very well by patients – they are also safer to use over long periods of time.

3. Many long-term health problems do not respond well to modern medicinal treatments – in these cases, herbal remedies are often more effective and

unlikely to cause dangerous side effects.

4. Herbal remedies are much more cost-effective – you can gather the ingredients on your own and do not have to go through an insurance company to get them.

5. Compared to prescription drugs, herbal remedies are much more widely available – there are many that you can even grow in your own home.

Note: It is important to keep in mind that herbal remedies may not act as quickly as prescription drugs or over-the-counter remedies. They are, however, healthier for your body in the long run and are less likely to cause harmful side effects.

Herbal Recipes for Health and Healing

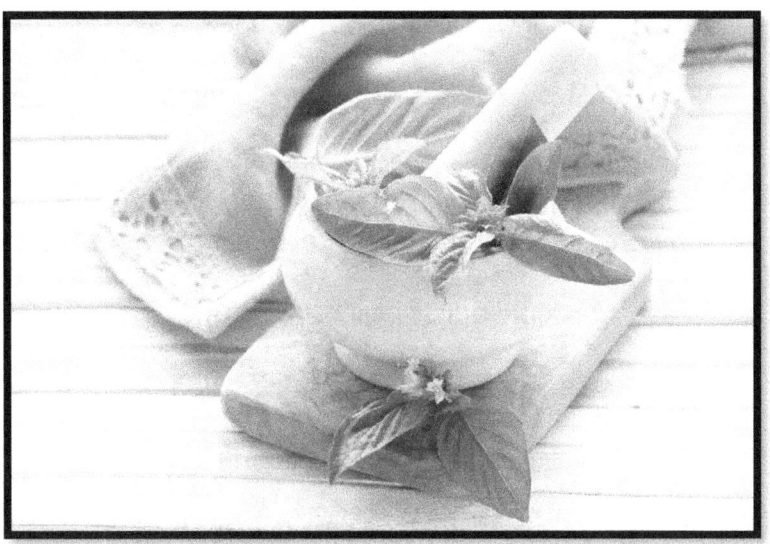

Recipes Included in this Book:

Dandelion Tea for Digestion

Calendula Tincture for Sore Gums

Comfrey Compress for Irritated Skin

Chamomile Poultice for Earache

Echinacea Tea for Cold/Flu

Antibacterial Healing Salve

Yarrow Tea for Cold and Flu

Goldenseal Antiseptic Poultice

Hawthorn Tonic

Calendula Tea for Sore Throat

Chamomile Wash for Burns and Boils

Comfrey Poultice for Bruises and Sprains

Hot Ginger Tea for Nausea

Yarrow Poultice to Stop Bleeding

Marshmallow Tea for Congestion

Mugwort Tincture for Stress Relief or Amenorrhea

Mullein Garlic Earache Compress

Nettle Tea for Bone and Joint Health

Peppermint Compress for Tension Headaches

St. John's Wort Tonic for Depression

Valerian Root Tea for Insomnia

Willow Bark Tea for Fever Reduction

Dandelion Tea for Digestion

Dandelion root is a natural diuretic and a gentle laxative that, when used to make tea, can help to regulate digestion. Drink this tea in the morning to encourage regularity or use it occasionally to relieve constipation. As an added bonus, this tea may help to rid your body of the bacteria and toxins that cause acne.

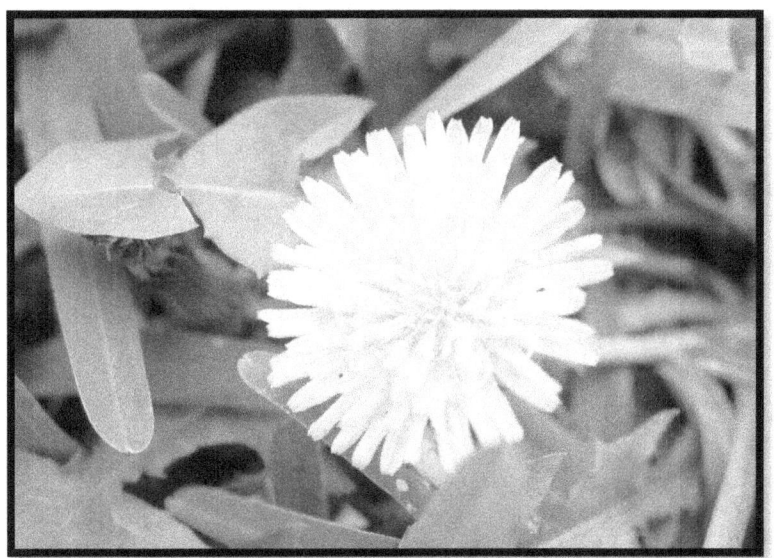

Ingredients:

8 ounces water

1 teaspoon chopped dandelion root

Instructions:

1. Combine the water and dandelion root in a small saucepan.
2. Bring the water to boil and let the dandelion root steep for 10 minutes.
3. Sweeten the tea with honey, if desired.
4. Enjoy daily in the morning for increased regularity in digestion.

Chamomile Poultice for Earache

While chamomile is most commonly used to make tea that encourages healthy sleep, it can also be used to reduce swelling and ease pain associated with a swollen jaw or earache. This recipe can be applied to clean muslin to create a compress that will help reduce swelling and relieve pain.

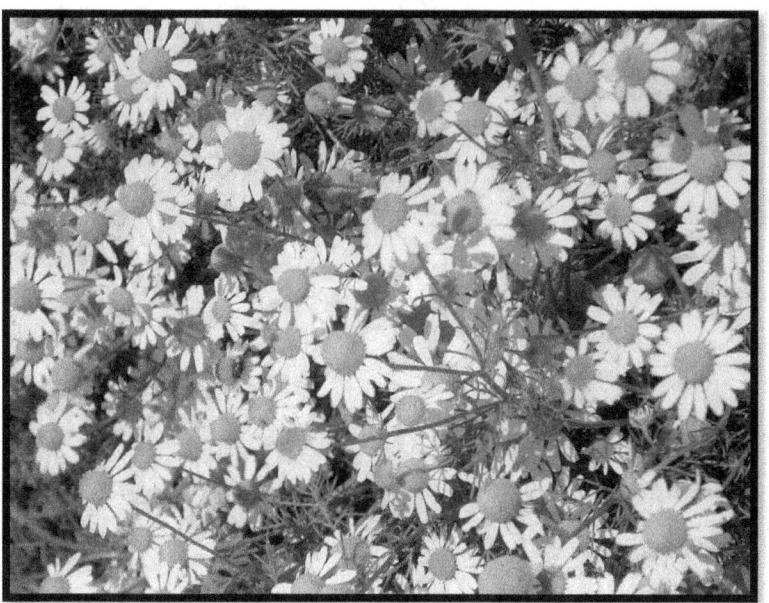

Ingredients:

½ cup dried chamomile flowers

Water, as needed

Muslin

Instructions:

1. Place the chamomile flowers in a heat proof bowl.
2. Pour the water into a small saucepan and bring to a boil then remove from heat and cool for 3 minutes.
3. Add enough boiled water to the bowl to cover the chamomile flowers.

4. Let the chamomile steep for 20 minutes, stirring it occasionally.

5. Transfer the mixture to a blender and blend on high speed until it forms a thick paste – add more water if needed a tablespoon at a time.

6. Apply the poultice to a piece of muslin and fold or layer it a few times.

7. Press the poultice-soaked muslin against your ear or jaw to reduce swelling and relieve pain.

Calendula Tincture for Sore Gums

The calendula flower has a number of medicinal properties and can be used to treat everything from sore throat to mouth ulcers. This tincture made from calendula flowers is specifically designed to treat sore gums and to heal mouth ulcers. You can also add a teaspoon of this tincture to warm water for a sore throat gargle.

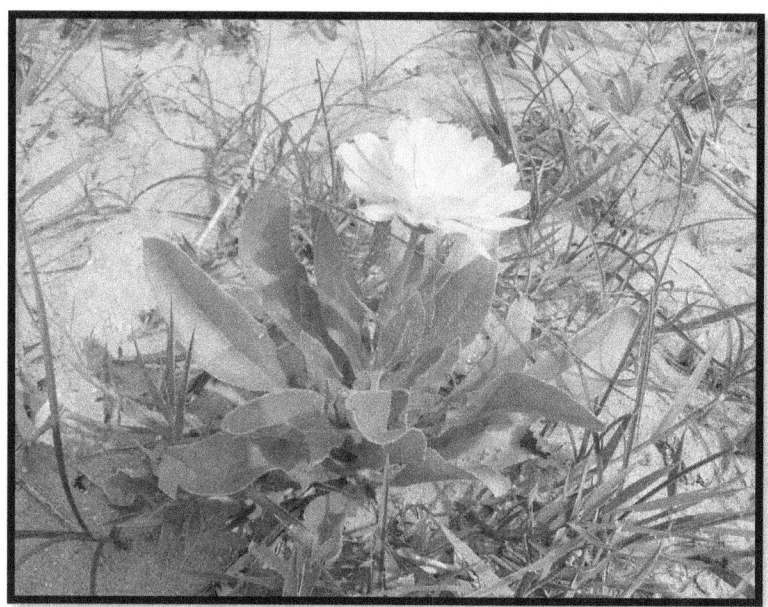

Ingredients:

½ cup dried calendula flowers, packed

4 ounces high-proof grain alcohol

1 ounce distilled water

Instructions:

1. Place the dried calendula flowers in a spice grinder and grind into a powder.
2. Measure out ¼ cup of the powder and set aside the rest for another recipe.
3. Transfer the powder to a glass jar and pour in the water and alcohol.

4. Shake the mixture well to saturate the powder then let it rest at room temperature for 14 days.

5. Shake the jar twice a day every day for two weeks then let rest for a full 24 hours.

6. Strain the mixture through a piece of fine cheesecloth and squeeze as much liquid from the flowers as you can.

7. Discard the solids and collect the liquid in a dark glass bottle.

8. Take 1 to 2ml of the tincture directly by mouth 3 to 4 times daily.

Valerian Root Tea for Insomnia

Valerian root has strong sedative properties but it doesn't lead to addiction and it doesn't put you in the kind of sleep that leaves you feeling groggy in the morning. For treatment of occasional insomnia, this valerian root tea is a great option.

Ingredients:

1 teaspoon dried valerian root

8 ounces boiling water

1 teaspoon fresh lemon juice

1 teaspoon honey

Instructions:

1. Place the valerian root in a large mug.
2. Pour in the hot water and let steep for 10 to 15 minutes.
3. Strain the liquid and discard the herb.
4. Stir in the honey and lemon juice then enjoy.

Comfrey Compress for Irritated Skin

The leaves of the comfrey plant are beneficial for healing wounds, moisturizing dry skin, soothing irritated skin and preventing or decreasing the appearance of scars. This compress made using a comfrey infusion has both anti-inflammatory and analgesic benefits that may help to treat everything from general skin irritation to conditions like psoriasis and eczema.

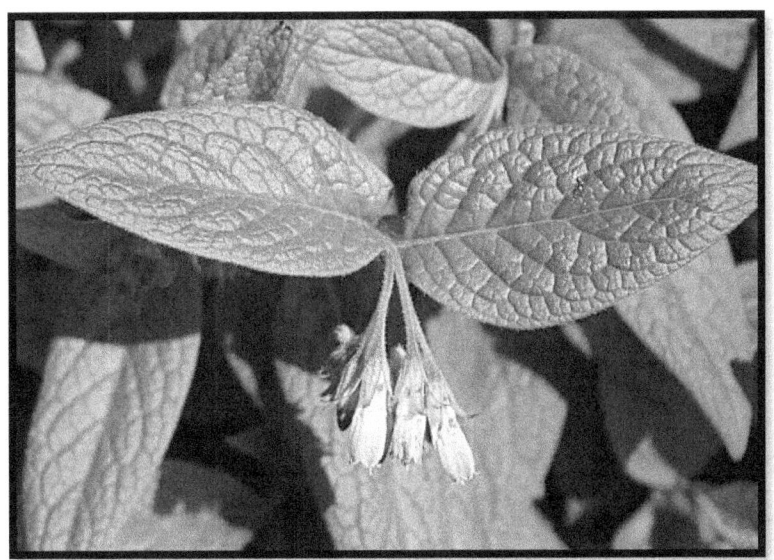

Ingredients:

1 cup dried comfrey leaf

½ cup finely chopped comfrey root

2 cups extra-virgin olive oil

Instructions:

1. Place the comfrey leaf and root in a glass jar.
2. Pour in the oil until the ingredients are completely covered then tightly cover with the lid.

3. Shake the jar until the ingredients are completely saturated then let rest at room temperature for 28 days.

4. Strain the mixture through a cheesecloth and discard the solids after squeezing out as much oil as possible.

5. To use the comfrey infusion, soak a clean cloth in the infusion and apply directly to the affected area.

Echinacea Tea for Cold/Flu

This Echinacea tea serves multiple purposes. It can be enjoyed daily to boost your immune system or you can start drinking it several times a day when you feel a cold coming on to reduce its longevity and to speed recovery. The addition of ginger to this recipe helps to reduce inflammation and gives the tea a more pleasant flavor.

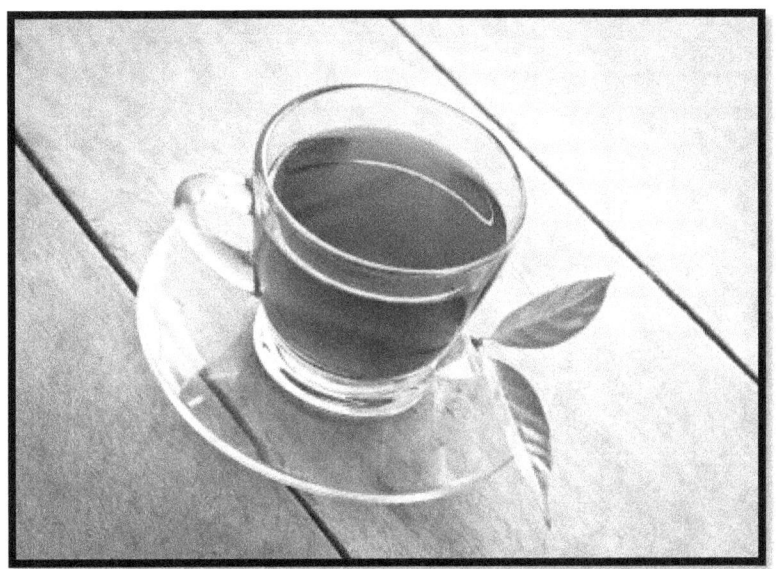

Ingredients:

1 teaspoon dried Echinacea

1 teaspoon fresh grated ginger

2 cups boiling water

1 teaspoon fresh lemon juice

1 teaspoon honey

Instructions:

1. Place the Echinacea and ginger in a large mug.
2. Pour in the boiling water and let steep for 15 minutes.
3. Stir in the lemon juice and honey.

4. Enjoy once daily for an immune system boost.

5. Drink the tea 2-3 times daily to stave off a cold.

Hawthorn Tonic

The berries of the hawthorn plant are commonly used to treat heart-related conditions. This hawthorn tincture can be used daily to improve heart health and stave off a heart attack by helping regulate blood pressure and improving blood flow through the arteries to the heart.

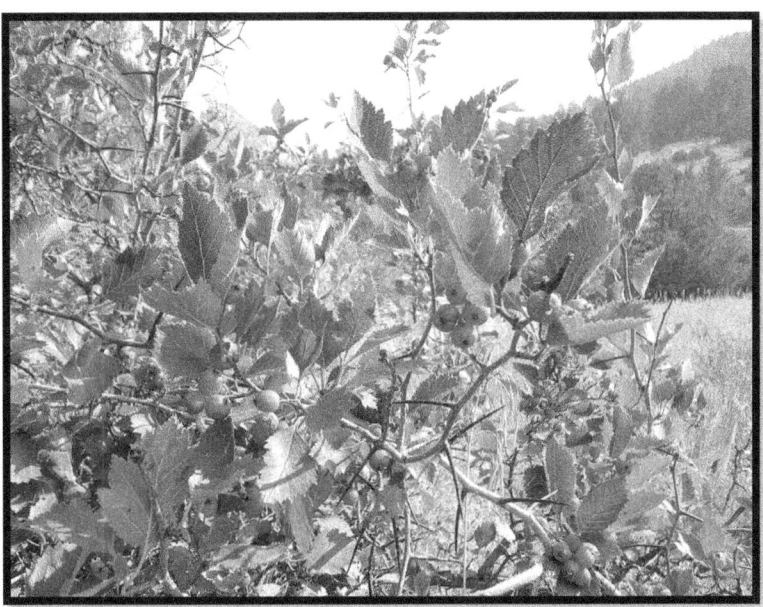

Ingredients:

1 cup dried hawthorn berries

2 cups high-proof brandy

Instructions:

1. Place the berries in a glass pint jar.
2. Pour in the brandy to cover the berries then screw the lid on tightly.
3. Store the jar in a cool, dark area for 2 to 4 weeks, shaking once daily.
4. Strain the liquid through a mesh strainer and discard the solids.
5. Pour the tincture into dark glass bottles.

6. Take 2 teaspoons by mouth daily for improved heart health.

Antibacterial Healing Salve

This homemade healing salve is made with several medicinal herbs, including Echinacea root, comfrey, calendula and yarrow. Use this salve in the same way that you would use Neosporin to treat cuts, burns, bruises, insect bites and other forms of skin irritation. Store the salve in small lip balm containers and keep one in your purse.

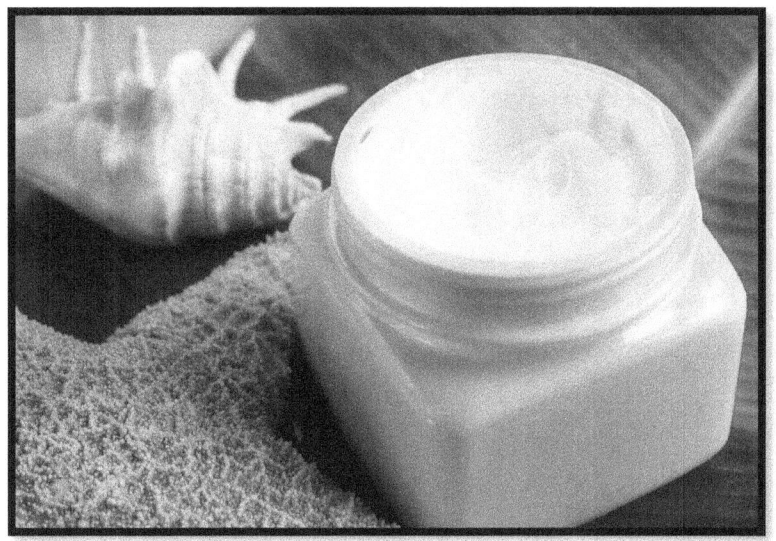

Ingredients:

2 cups extra-virgin olive oil

2 ½ tablespoons comfrey leaf

1 ½ tablespoons plantain leaf

1 tablespoon dried calendula flowers

1 teaspoon Echinacea root

1 teaspoon dried yarrow flowers

¼ cup beeswax pellets

½ teaspoon vitamin E oil

Instructions:

1. Pour the olive oil into a double boiler over low heat.
2. Stir in the herbs until they are fully saturated then let steep for 3 hours, stirring occasionally.
3. When the oil is very green in color, strain out the herbs using a fine mesh or cheesecloth, squeezing as much oil out as you can.
4. Add the infused oil back to the double boiler and stir in the beeswax.
5. When the beeswax is melted, remove from heat and whisk in the vitamin E oil.
6. Pour the mixture into small jars or lip balm containers and cool to room temperature.
7. Store in a cool, dry place and apply directly to clean skin as needed.

Yarrow Tea for Cold and Flu

While yarrow is primarily known for its ability to stop bleeding, it can also be used to make a tea that helps your body to expel toxins and to reduce fever. Unfortunately, this herb has a strong bitter taste, so you may need to sweeten the tea with honey.

Ingredients:

2 teaspoons dried yarrow

1 ½ cups boiling water

1 tablespoon honey

Instructions:

1. Place the yarrow in a large mug.
2. Pour in the boiling water and let steep for 15 minutes.
3. Stir in the honey and enjoy immediately.

Goldenseal Antiseptic Poultice

The goldenseal herb has a wide variety of medicinal properties – it can be used to treat skin infections as well as mouth ulcers. This herb can also be used in poultice form as a topical antiseptic for minor cuts, scrapes and abrasions. The addition of comfrey to this poultice helps to further speed healing.

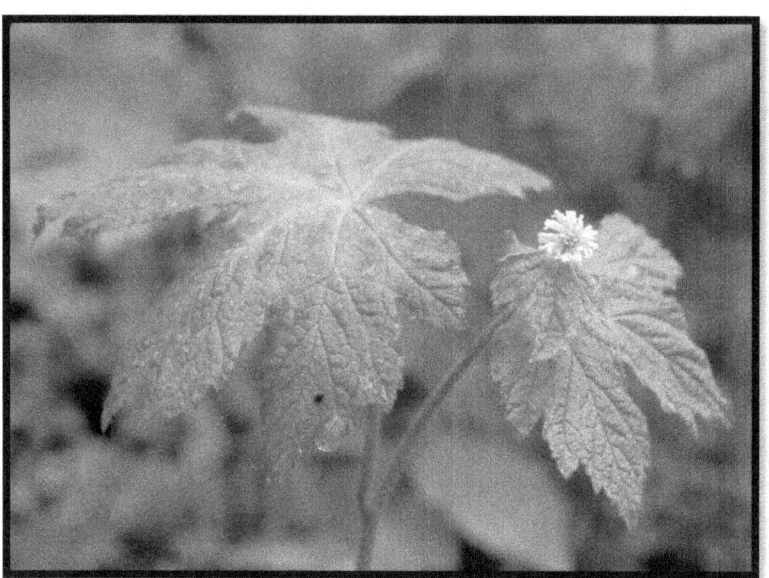

Ingredients:

2 tablespoons dried goldenseal

1 tablespoon dried comfrey

Warm water, as needed

Gauze bandages

Instructions:

1. Place the dried herbs in a small bowl.
2. Grind the herbs by hand or use a spice grinder.
3. Add a small amount of water to the powdered herbs, stirring to form a thick paste.

4. Spread the paste on the affected area and cover lightly with gauze.

5. Leave the poultice on until it dries out then rinse the area with warm water.

Calendula Tea for Sore Throat

This calendula tea is an excellent all-natural treatment for sore throat. Enjoy this tea daily as needed or use it as a gargle to soothe your throat. Alternatively, you can apply this tea directly to your skin to soothe and heal rashes or insect bites. This tea is gentle enough to be used for children – it may also help soothe an upset stomach.

Ingredients:

2 teaspoons dried calendula flowers

8 ounces water

Instructions:

1. Combine the water and calendula flowers in a small saucepan.
2. Bring the water to boil and let the calendula steep for 10 minutes.
3. Sweeten the tea with honey, if desired.
4. Enjoy daily as needed to soothe a sore throat.

Chamomile Wash for Burns and Boils

When combined with lavender and tea tree essential oils, chamomile essential oil makes for a very effective skin wash. This wash can be used to treat cuts and scrapes or to relieve the pain and swelling associated with burns and boils.

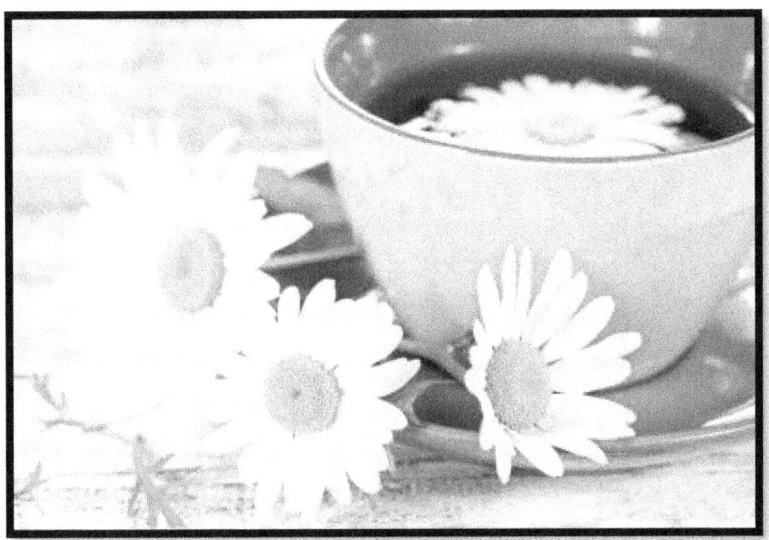

Ingredients:

2 cups hot water

3 drops chamomile essential oil

2 drops lavender essential oil

2 drops tea tree essential oil

Instructions:

1. Pour the water into a bowl.
2. Add the essential oils and stir gently.
3. Stir well then saturate a clean cloth in the mixture.
4. Wring out the excess moisture from the cloth.
5. Apply the cloth to the affected skin area, using firm pressure.

6. Repeat the treatment twice daily as needed.

Yarrow Poultice to Stop Bleeding

Yarrow is sometimes referred to using the nickname "nosebleed" due to its powerful ability to stop bleeding. This yarrow poultice can help to stop even profuse bleeding when applied with firm compression. In the case of open wounds, make sure to keep several layers of gauze between the poultice and the wound.

Ingredients:

2 tablespoons dried yarrow leaf

Warm water, as needed

Gauze bandages

Instructions:

1. Grind the yarrow with a mortar and pestle into a fine powder.
2. As an alternative, grind the yarrow in a spice grinder.
3. Add a small amount of water to the powdered herb, stirring to form a thick paste.
4. Spread the paste on a piece of gauze and fold it over once or twice.
5. Apply the gauze compress to the affected area and apply pressure until the bleeding stops.
6. Leave the poultice on until it dries out then rinse the area with warm water.

Comfrey Poultice for Bruises and Sprains

Earlier in this book you received a recipe for a comfrey infusion that can be applied directly to the skin as a treatment for irritation. This poultice uses the same ingredients but is made using a hot rather than a cold infusion method. This comfrey poultice can be applied to bruises and sprains to facilitate the production of new cells, thereby speeding the healing process.

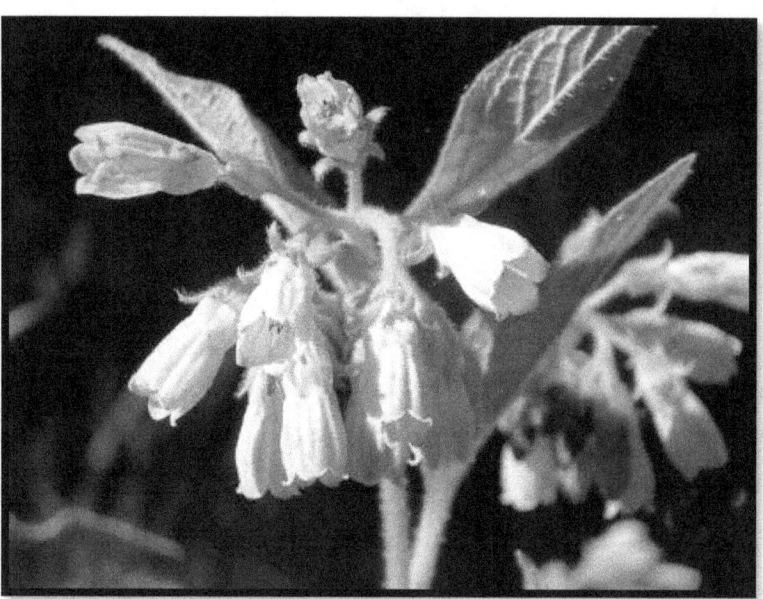

Ingredients:

½ cup dried comfrey root, finely chopped

Water, as needed

Gauze bandages

Instructions:

1. Place the comfrey root in a heat proof bowl.
2. Pour the water into a small saucepan and bring to a boil then remove from heat and cool for 3 minutes.
3. Add enough boiled water to the bowl to cover the comfrey.

4. Let the comfrey root steep for 20 minutes, stirring it occasionally.
5. Transfer the mixture to a blender and blend on high speed until it forms a thick paste – add more water if needed a tablespoon at a time.
6. Spread a layer of the poultice on a gauze bandage and apply to the affected area.
7. Wrap the area in clean gauze bandages and leave in place overnight or until the poultice has dried.

Marshmallow Tea for Congestion

Marshmallow root provides valuable mucilage benefits, which is particularly beneficial for relieving sinus pressure and congestion. This marshmallow root tea is easy to make and can be combined with mullein for extra power against persistent cough and cold.

Ingredients:

1 tablespoon chopped marshmallow root

1 teaspoon dried peppermint leaf

8 ounces hot water

Instructions:

1. Place the marshmallow root and peppermint leaf in a mug.
2. Pour in the hot water and let steep for 10 minutes.
3. Strain the mixture and discard the solids.
4. Enjoy the tea 2 to 3 times daily as needed.

Hot Ginger Tea for Nausea

Ginger root has a hot and spicy flavor that works very well in tea. Additionally, it provides a number of medicinal benefits, such as improving digestion and soothing digestive upset. Drink this tea to calm nausea associated with morning sickness, motion sickness, or chemotherapy treatments.

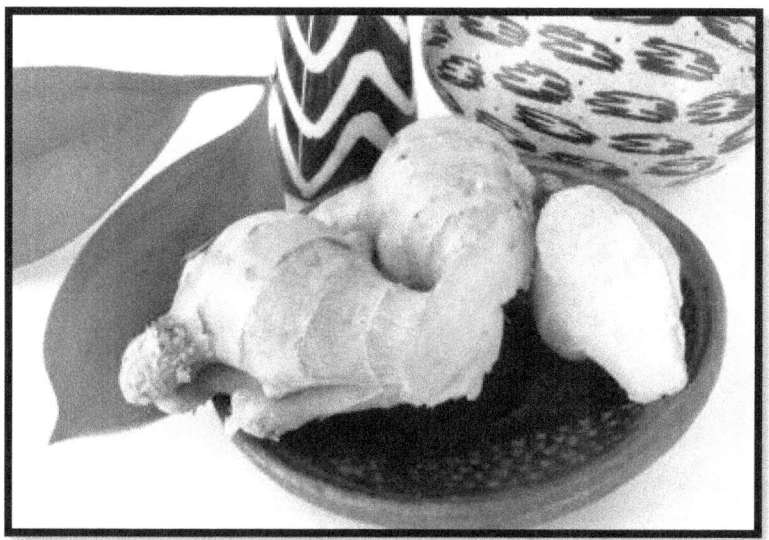

Ingredients:

1 tablespoon fresh grated ginger

Pinch ground cinnamon

2 cups water

1 tablespoon fresh lemon juice

1 to 2 teaspoons honey

Instructions:

1. Place the ginger and cinnamon in a small saucepan.
2. Pour in the water and bring to a boil.
3. Turn off the heat and let the mixture steep, covered, for 10 minutes.

4. Strain the liquid and discard the solids.

5. Stir in the lemon juice and honey then enjoy immediately.

Mugwort Tincture for Stress Relief or Amenorrhea

Mugwort is a powerful herb that has natural stimulant properties. These properties make it a good treatment for both depression and amenorrhea in women. To achieve the maximum benefit from this tincture, use it daily.

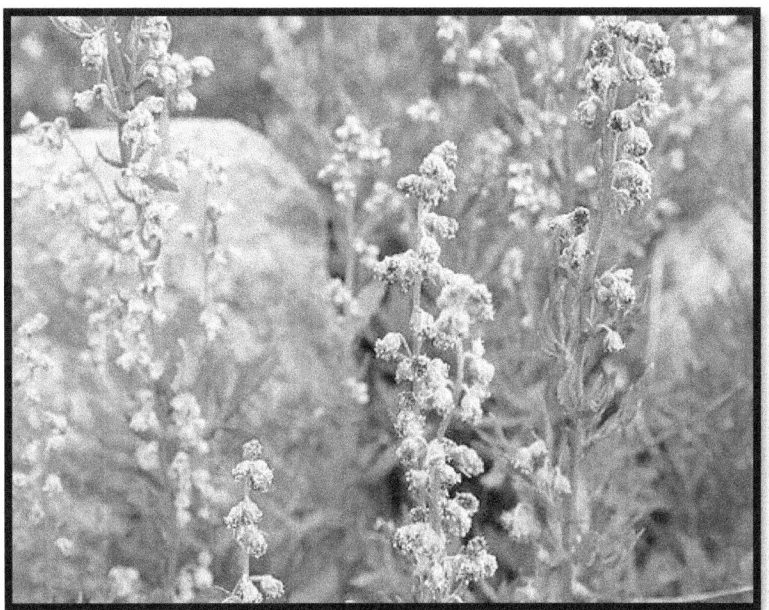

Ingredients:

½ cup dried mugwort

4 ounces high-proof vodka

1 ounce distilled water

Instructions:

1. Place the dried mugwort in a spice grinder and grind into a powder.
2. Measure out ¼ cup of the powder and set aside the rest for another recipe.
3. Transfer the powder to a glass jar and pour in the water and vodka.
4. Shake the mixture well to saturate the powder then let it rest at room temperature for 14 days.

5. Shake the jar twice a day every day for two weeks then let rest for a full 24 hours.

6. Strain the mixture through a piece of fine cheesecloth and squeeze as much liquid from the mugwort as you can.

7. Discard the solids and collect the liquid in a dark glass bottle.

8. Take 1 to 2ml of the tincture directly by mouth twice daily.

Mullein Garlic Earache Compress

This mullein garlic earache compress will come in very handy if you have a child who is prone to earaches. Not only is this compress easy to prepare, but it is gentle enough that you never have to worry about negative side effects for your child.

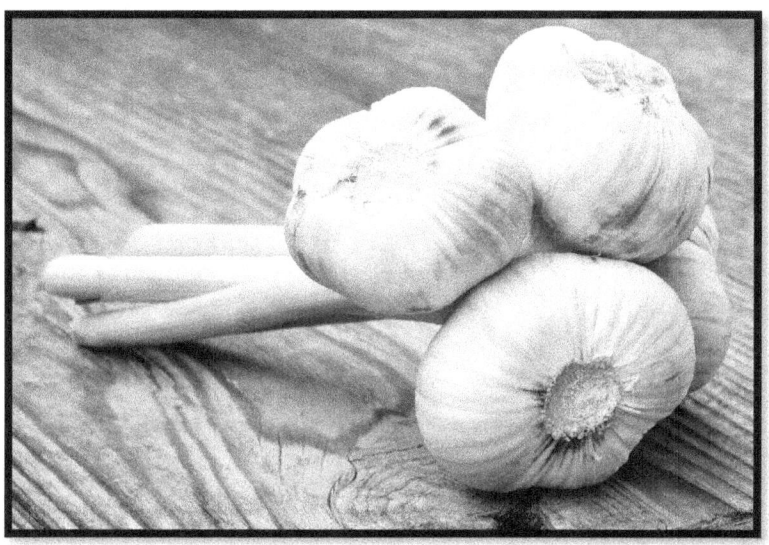

Ingredients:

1 head garlic, peeled

1 ounce dried mullein flowers

2 cups extra-virgin olive oil

Instructions:

1. Combine the ingredients in a small saucepan and stir well.
2. Simmer over low heat for 1 hour.
3. Strain the mixture and discard the solids and cool to room temperature.
4. Store in the refrigerator for up to 2 years.
5. To use the mixture, add a few drops to a spoon and heat with a match.
6. Be careful not to make it too hot.

7. Soak up the oil with a cotton ball and apply it directly to the ear.

8. Repeat the treatment 3 to 5 times daily.

Nettle Tea for Bone and Joint Health

When you think of nettles, you probably picture a prickly, nuisance plant. In reality, this plant is a strong medicinal herb that can help to soothe the pain associated with bone and joint problems like arthritis and gout. This tea has natural anti-inflammatory properties that, when enjoyed daily, can relieve bone and joint issues. Drinking this tea daily may help to relieve the pain of arthritis and other joint health problems.

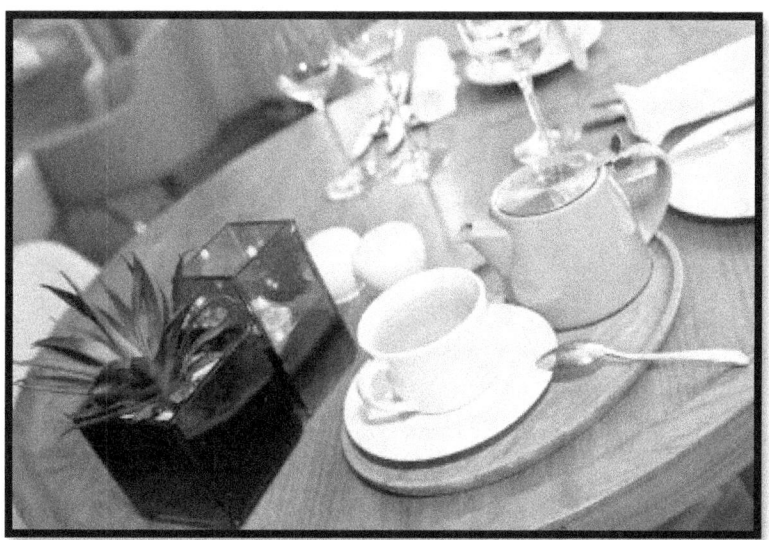

Ingredients:

1 cup fresh nettle leaves

4 cups water

1 tablespoon honey

Instructions:

1. Wash the nettle leaves well then place them in a large saucepan.
2. Add the water and bring to a boil.
3. Simmer, covered, for 15 minutes then strain the liquid, squeezing the leaves, and discard the leaves.

4. Stir in the honey and pour into a mug to serve.

Peppermint Compress for Tension Headaches

Peppermint is not only a flavorful and aromatic herb, but it also contains valuable medicinal benefits. This peppermint compress, for example, is a great way to relieve the pain and pressure of tension headaches.

Ingredients:

Cold water

Peppermint essential oil

Clean cloth

Instructions:

1. Fill a bowl with cold water and add a few drops of peppermint essential oil.
2. Soak the cloth in the water then wring out the extra moisture.
3. Apply the compress to the back of the neck or forehead to relieve tension headaches.

St. John's Wort Tonic for Depression

St. John's Wort is a great herbal remedy for mood problems like depression and anxiety. When used in tea, St. John's Wort can act as a general tonic for the nervous system. This tonic can be taken daily to help relieve the symptoms of anxiety and depression.

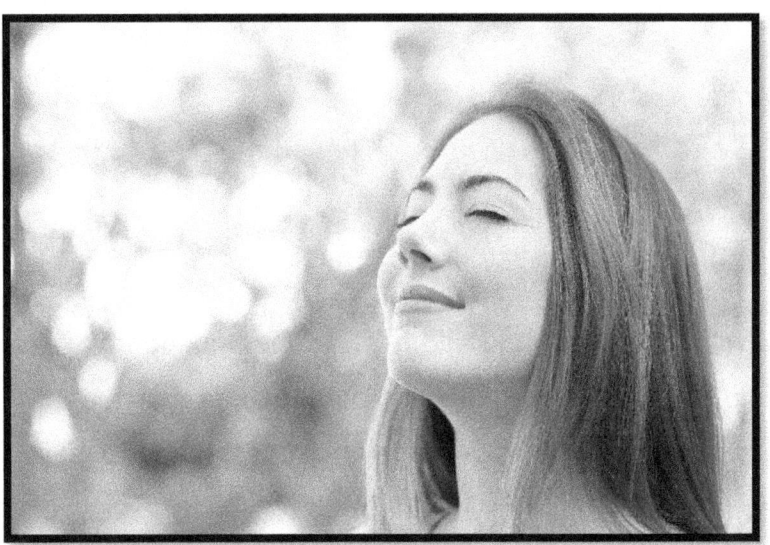

Ingredients:

3 ounces dried St. John's Wort

8 ounces 100-proof vodka

Instructions:

1. Place the St. John's Wort in a glass jar and pour in the vodka.
2. Shake the mixture well to saturate the herb then let it rest at room temperature for 14 days.
3. Shake the jar twice a day every day for two weeks then let rest for a full 24 hours.
4. Strain the mixture through a piece of fine cheesecloth and squeeze as much liquid from the herb as you can.

5. Discard the solids and collect the liquid in a dark glass bottle.

6. Take 1 to 2ml daily directly by mouth.

Willow Bark Tincture for Fever Reduction

As you read earlier in this book, willow bark has many of the same benefits as aspirin. This willow bark tincture can help to reduce the pain and inflammation associated with high fever, and it can be taken daily to prevent heart attack.

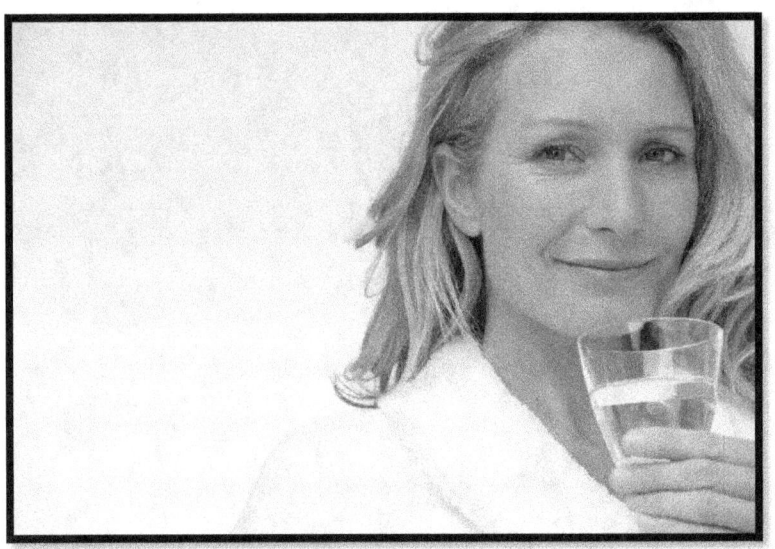

Ingredients:

½ cup dried chopped willow bark

4 ounces high-proof vodka

1 ounce distilled water

Instructions:

1. Place the dried willow bark in a spice grinder and grind into a powder.
2. Measure out ¼ cup of the powder and set aside the rest for another recipe.
3. Transfer the powder to a glass jar and pour in the water and vodka.
4. Shake the mixture well to saturate the powder then let it rest at room temperature for 14 days.
5. Shake the jar twice a day every day for two weeks then let rest for a full 24 hours.

6. Strain the mixture through a piece of fine cheesecloth and squeeze as much liquid from the bark as you can.

7. Discard the solids and collect the liquid in a dark glass bottle.

8. Take 1 to 2ml of the tincture directly by mouth twice daily to prevent heart attack or to treat fever.

Conclusion

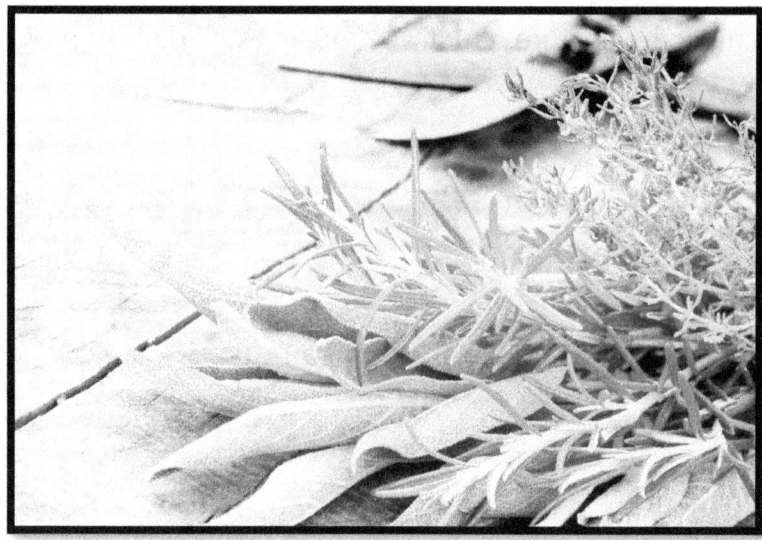

After reading this book, you should have a firm understanding of what medicinal herbs are and how they can be used. In addition to learning the benefits of natural herbal remedies in general, you have also received detailed profiles of twenty of the top medicinal herbs. Use these herbs in the recipes provided in this book to treat common health problems as an alternative to drugs and over-the-counter remedies. You may be surprised to find that they work just as well, or even better!

I Need Your Help!

Please take a minute out of your busy schedule to leave a review.

Your review will let readers know what to expect and what you liked about this book. I am looking forward to reading your review.

Thank you so much for your feedback!

How to Submit a Review

To submit a review:

1. Make sure you are signed in.
2. Hover over **Your Account** in the upper right hand corner.
3. Click on **Your Orders**.
4. Click on **Digital Orders**.
5. Click **Write a customer review** in the Customer Reviews section.
6. Rate the item and write your review.
7. Click **Submit**.

How to submit a review from your Kindle device

Please follow the link below for instructions.

http://www.dummies.com/how-to/content/posting-an-amazon-book-review-from-your-kindle.html

www.ingramcontent.com/pod-product-compliance
Lightning Source LLC
Chambersburg PA
CBHW080610290526

45790CB00007B/2720